The Essential Keto Diet Cookbook

Super Tasty Keto Recipes For Any Occasion And For Any Budget

Elena Harrison

Table of Contents

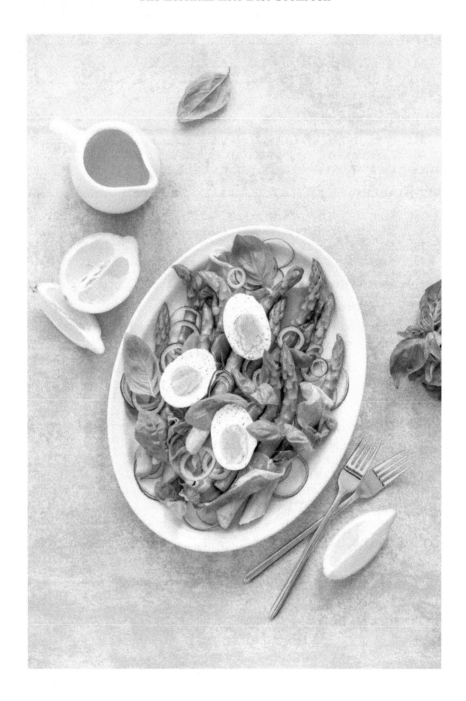

INTRODUCTION

The ketogenic diet has been highly praised and praised for the benefits of weight loss. This high-fat, low-carb diet has been shown to be extremely healthy overall. It really makes your body burn fat, like a talking machine. Public figures appreciate it too. But the question is, how does ketosis enhance weight loss? The following is a detailed picture of the ketosis and weight loss process.

Some people consider ketosis to be abnormal. Although it has been approved by many nutritionists and doctors. many people still disapprove of it. The misconceptions are due to the myths that have spread around the ketogenic diet.

Once your body is out of glucose, it automatically depends on stored fat. It is also important to understand that carbohydrates produce glucose and once you start a low carbohydrate diet, you will also be able to lower your glucose levels. Then your body will produce fuel through fat, instead of carbohydrates, that is, glucose.

The process of accumulating fat through fat is known as ketosis, and once your body enters this state, it becomes extremely effective at burning unwanted fat. Also, since glucose levels are low during the ketogenic diet, your body achieves many other health benefits.

A ketogenic diet is not only beneficial for weight loss, but it also helps improve your overall health in a positive way. Unlike all other diet plans, which focus on reducing calorie intake, ketogenic focuses on putting your body in a natural metabolic state, that is, ketosis. The only factor that makes this diet questionable is that this nature of metabolism is not very well thought out. By getting tattoos on your body regularly, your body will quickly burn stored fat, leading to great weight loss.

Now the question arises. How does ketosis affect the human body?

However, this phase does not last more than 2-3 days. This is the time it takes for the human body to enter the ketosis phase. Once you get in, you won't have any side effects.

You should also start gradually reducing your calorie and carbohydrate intake. The most common mistake dietitians make is that they tend to start eliminating everything from their diet at the same time. This is where the problem arises. The human body will react extremely negatively when you limit everything at once. You must start gradually. Read this guide to learn more about how to approach the ketogenic diet after 50.

Most fats are good and essential for our health so there are essential fatty acids and essential amino acids (proteins). Fat is the most efficient form of energy, and each gram contains about 9 calories. This more than doubles the amount of carbohydrates and protein (both have 4 calories per gram).

When you eat a lot of fat and protein and significantly reduce carbohydrates, your body adjusts and converts the fat and protein, as well as the fat that it has stored, into ketones or ketones, for energy. This metabolic process is called ketosis. This is where the ketogen in the ketogenic diet comes from.

BREAKFAST

1. Eggs and Bell Peppers

Preparation time: 5 minutes

Cooking time: 20 minutes

Servings: 4

Ingredients:

- 1 red bell pepper, cut into strips
- 1 green bell pepper, cut into strips
- 1 orange bell pepper, cut into strips
- 4 eggs, whisked
- Salt and black pepper to the taste
- 2 tablespoons mozzarella, shredded
- Cooking spray

Directions:

1. In a bowl, mix the eggs with all the bell peppers, salt and pepper and toss.
2. Heat up the air fryer at 350 degrees F, grease it with cooking spray, pour the eggs mixture, spread well, sprinkle the mozzarella on top and cook for 20 minutes.
3. Divide between plates and serve for breakfast.

Nutrition: Calories 229 Fat 13 Fiber 3 carbohydrates 4 Protein 7

2. <u>Cauliflower Casserole</u>

Preparation time: 5 minutes

Cooking time: 20 minutes

Servings: 4

Ingredients:

- 2 cups cauliflower florets, separated
- 4 eggs, whisked
- 1 teaspoon sweet paprika
- 2 tablespoons butter, melted
- A pinch of salt and black pepper

Directions:

1. Heat up your air fryer at 320 degrees F, grease with the butter, add cauliflower florets on the bottom, then add eggs whisked with paprika, salt and pepper, toss and cook for 20 minutes.
2. Divide between plates and serve for breakfast.

Nutrition: Calories 240 Fat 9 Fiber 2 carbohydrates 4 Protein 8

KETO BREAD

3. Great flavor cheese bread with the added kick of pimento olives.

Preparation Time: 5 Minutes

Cooking Time: 3 Hours

Servings: 1 Loaf

Ingredients

- cup water room temperature
- 4 tsp. sugar
- 3/4 tsp. salt
- 1 ¼ cups shredded sharp cheddar cheese
- cups bread flour
- tsp. active dry yeast
- 3/4 cup pimiento olives, drained and sliced

Direction:

1. Add all ingredients except olives to machine pan.
2. Select basic bread setting.
3. At prompt before second knead, mix in olives.

Nutrition: 124 Calories, 4 g total fat (2 g sat. fat), 9 mg chol, 299 mg sodium, 19 g carb. 1 fiber, 5 g protein

4. Ricotta Chive Bread

Preparation Time: 5 minutes

Cooking Time: 3 hours

Servings: 1 loaf

Ingredients

- cup lukewarm water
- 1/3 cup whole or part-skim ricotta cheese
- 1 ½ tsp. salt
- 1 tablespoon granulated sugar
- cups bread flour
- 1/2 cup chopped chives
- ½ tsp. instant yeast

Direction:

1. Add ingredients to bread machine pan except dried fruit.
2. Choose basic bread setting and light/medium crust.

Nutrition: 92 Calories, 0 g total fat (0 g sat. fat), 2 mg chol, 207 mg sodium, 17 g carb. 1 fiber, 3 g protein

5. Red Hot Cinnamon Bread

Preparation Time: 5 minutes

Cooking Time: 3 hours

Servings: 1 loaf

Ingredients

- 1/4 cup lukewarm water
- 1/2 cup lukewarm milk
- 1/4 cup softened butter
- 2 ¼ tsp. instant yeast
- ¼ tsp. salt
- 1/4 cup sugar
- 1 tsp. vanilla
- 1 large egg, lightly beaten
- cups all-purpose flour
- 1/2 cup Cinnamon Red Hot candies

Direction:

1. Add ingredients to bread machine pan except candy.
2. Choose dough setting.
3. After cycle is over, turn dough out into bowl and cover, let rise for 45 minutes to one hour.
4. Gently punch down dough and shape into a rectangle.
5. Knead in the cinnamon candies in 1/3 at a t time.
6. Shape the dough into a loaf and place in a greased or parchment lined loaf pan.

7. Tent the pan loosely with lightly greased plastic wrap, and allow a second rise for 40-50 minutes.

8. Preheat oven 350 degrees.

9. Bake 30-40 minutes.

10. Remove and cool on wire rack before slicing.

Nutrition: 207 Calories, 6.9 g total fat (4.1 g sat. fat), 28 mg chol, 317 mg sodium, 30 g carb. 1 fiber, 4.6 g protein 62.Cheddar Olive Loaf

6. Wild Rice Cranberry Bread

Preparation Time: 5 minutes

Cooking Time: 3 hours

Servings: 1 loaf

Ingredients

- ¼ cup water
- 1/4 cup skim milk powder
- 1 ¼ tsp. salt
- tablespoon liquid honey
- 1 tablespoon extra-virgin olive oil
- cup all-purpose flour
- 3/4 cup cooked wild rice
- 1/4 cup pine nuts
- 3/4 tsp. celery seeds
- 1/8 tsp. freshly ground black pepper
- 1 tsp. bread machine or instant yeast
- 2/3 cup dried cranberries

Direction:

1. Add all ingredients to machine pan except the cranberries.
2. Place pan into the oven chamber.
3. Select basic bread setting.
4. At the signal to add ingredients, add in the cranberries.

Nutrition: 225 Calories, 7.8 g total fat (1.2 g sat. fat), 5 mg chol, 182 mg sodium, 33 g carb. 1 fiber, 6.7 g protein

7. Sauerkraut Rye Bread

Preparation Time: 5 minutes

Cooking Time: 3 hours

Servings: 1 loaf

Ingredients

- cup sauerkraut – rinsed and drained
- 3/4 cup warm water
- 1 ½ tablespoons molasses
- 1 ½ tablespoons butter
- 1 ½ tablespoons brown sugar
- 1 tsp. caraway seed
- 1 ½ tsp. salt
- 1 cup rye flour
- cups bread flour
- 1 ½ tsp. active dry yeast

Direction:

1. Add all ingredients to machine pan.
2. Select basic bread setting.

Nutrition: 74 Calories, 1.8 g total fat (0 g sat. fat), 4 mg chol, 411 mg sodium, 12 g carb. 1 fiber, 1.8 g protein

8. <u>Cheese Cauliflower Broccoli Bread</u>

Preparation Time: 10 minutes

Cooking Time: 3 hours

Servings: 1 loaf

Ingredients

- 1/4 cup water
- 4 tablespoons oil
- egg white
- 1 tsp. lemon juice
- 2/3 cup grated cheddar cheese
- Tablespoons green onion
- 1/2 cup broccoli, chopped
- 1/2 cup cauliflower, chopped
- 1/2 tsp. lemon-pepper seasoning
- cup bread flour
- 1 tsp. regular or quick-rising yeast

Direction:

1. Add all ingredients to machine pan.
2. Select basic bread setting.

Nutrition: 156 Calories, 7.4 g total fat (2.2 g sat. fat), 8 mg chol, 56 mg sodium, 17 g carb. 0 fiber, 4.9 g protein

9. <u>Orange Cappuccino Bread</u>

Preparation Time: 10 Minutes

Cooking Time: 3 Hours

Servings: 1 Loaf

Ingredients

- cup water

- 1 tablespoon instant coffee granules

- tablespoons butter or margarine, softened

- 1 tsp. grated orange peel

- cups Bread flour

- 2 tablespoons dry milk

- 1/4 cup sugar

- 1 ¼ tsp. salt

- 2 ¼ tsp. bread machine or quick active dry yeast

Direction:

1. Add all ingredients to machine pan.

2. Select basic bread setting.

Nutrition: 155 Calories, 2 g total fat (1 g sat. fat), 5 mg chol, 270 mg sodium, 31 g carb. 1 fiber, 4 g protein

10. Celery Bread

Preparation Time: 10 Minutes

Cooking Time: 3 Hours

Servings: 1 Loaf

Ingredients

- (10 oz.) can cream of celery soup
- tablespoons low-fat milk, heated
- 1 tablespoon vegetable oil
- 1 ¼ tsp. celery, garlic, or onion salt
- 3/4 cup celery, fresh/slice thin
- 1 tablespoon celery leaves, fresh, chopped -optional
- 1 egg
- cups bread flour
- 1/4 tsp. sugar
- 1/4 tsp. ginger
- 1/2 cup quick-cooking oats
- 2 tablespoons gluten
- 2 tsp. celery seeds
- 1 package active dry yeast

Direction:

1. Add all ingredients to machine pan.
2. Select basic bread setting.

Nutrition: 73 Calories, 3.6 g total fat (0 g sat. fat), 55 mg chol, 186 mg sodium, 8 g carb. 0 fiber, 2.6 g protein

11. Anise Almond Bread

Preparation Time: 10 minutes

Cooking Time: 3 hours

Servings: 1 loaf

Ingredients:

- 3/4 cup water
- or 1/4 cup egg substitute
- 1/4 cup butter or margarine, softened
- 1/4 cup sugar
- 1/2 tsp. salt
- cup bread flour
- 1 tsp. anise seed
- tsp. active dry yeast
- 1/2 cup almonds, chopped small

Direction:

1. Add all ingredients to machine pan except almonds.
2. Select basic bread setting.
3. After prompt, add almonds.

Nutrition: 78 Calories, 4 g total fat (1 g sat. fat), 4 mg chol, 182 mg sodium, 7 g carb. 0 fiber, 3 g protein

12. Cottage Cheese Bread

Preparation Time: 10 Minutes

Cooking Time: 3 Hours

Servings: 1 Loaf

Ingredients

- 1/2 cup water
- cup cottage cheese
- tablespoons margarine
- 1 egg
- 1 tablespoon white sugar
- 1/4 tsp. baking soda
- 1 tsp. salt
- cups bread flour
- 2 ½ tsp. active dry yeast

Direction:

1. Add all ingredients to machine pan. Use the order suggested by manufacturer.
2. Select basic bread setting.
3. Tip: If dough is too sticky, add up to ½ cup more flour.

Nutrition: 171 Calories, 3.6 g total fat (1 g sat. fat), 18 mg chol, 234 mg sodium, 26 g carb. 1 fiber, 7.3 g protein

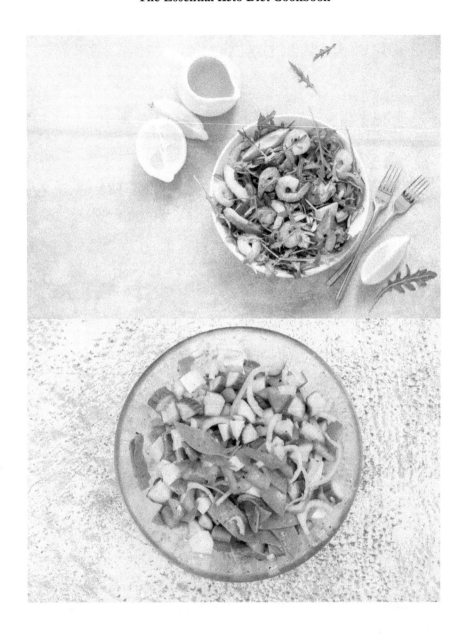

KETO PASTA

13. Bacon Herb Spaghetti Squash "Pasta" Salad

Preparation Time: 15 minutes

Cooking time: 32 minutes

Servings: 4

Ingredients:

- 1 spaghetti squash.
- 3 tbsp. bacon oil or lard.
- 1/2 tsp. raw salt.
- 1/2 tsp. dried out thyme.
- 1/4 tsp. black pepper (omit if desired).
- 1/2 tsp. celery salt or dried out marjoram for AIP.
- 1/4 tsp. ground dried out the sage.
- 1/2 cup fresh oregano, chopped.
- 3/4 to 1 cup sliced cooked bacon (if you can get smoked hog dewlaps, those are also better!).

Directions:

1. Preheat oven to 350F.
2. Slice spaghetti squash in half lengthwise using a sharp blade. Dig as well as dispose of seeds.

3. Separate bacon grease into half and place it in the scooped out holes. Split dry flavorings in half and spread uniformly over the cut fifty percent.

4. Place squash halves reduced side up in a glass recipe as well as include 1/4 -1/2-inch water to the bottom of the meal.

5. Cover with an ovenproof cover or foil and bake for about 30-40 mins, depending on just how large your own is. If you don't have pre-cooked bacon, lay slices in a solitary layer on a cookie sheet with a rim and bake while the squash is cooking. Depending on how thick the bacon is, it will probably require you to cook for 10-20 mins.

6. Once it is done to your liking, get rid of, allow trendy, then cut coarsely.

7. When the spaghetti squash is done, get rid of the oven. Once it is cool enough to take care of, remove the squash shreds using two forks and also place in a big bowl.

8. Mix in the chopped fresh oregano and bacon. Cover and cool in the fridge for several hrs until cooled down throughout.

9. Optional: Add numerous ounces of leftover shredded chicken (or other meat) to make it a full dish for a picnic or jam-packed lunch.

10. Served chilled. However, you can take it when it is hot if that is fine with you. Simply reheat in the stove for some mins till warmed enough. Season with salt or pepper!

Nutrition: Calories: 324 Sugar: 2 g Fat: 32 g Carbohydrates: 2 g Fiber: 3 g Protein: 54 g.

14. Zucchini Noodle Bolognese

Preparation Time: 15 minutes

Cooking time: 32 minutes

Servings: 4

Ingredients:

- 6 medium zucchini
- 1/2 pound light Italian sausage (bulk or coverings removed).
- 1 tablespoon avocado oil (or chosen cooking oil).
- 1/8 cup water.
- 1 orange bell pepper, seeded and also diced.
- 6 ramps (or 1 small diced onion + 2-3 cloves of garlic).
- 1 extra pound pearl or roma tomatoes.
- Sea salt.
- Black pepper.

Directions:

1. Clean ramps. Remove and discard roots. Chop the fallen leaves off over the pink stems and. DO NOT discard the leaves

2. Chop them up very well, keep 2 tablespoons to garnish. Chop the ramps.

3. Peel zucchini. Spiralize zucchini or use a mandolin and also pieces zucchini to form "lengthy noodles." Place them in a colander and also spray with concerning a teaspoon of sea salt.

4. Heat oil in a frying pan on medium-high heat. Place cut ramps and also leaves in the skillet in addition to the sausage, bell

pepper, salt, and pepper to taste. Cook for 5 minutes up until sausage is practically cooked through.

5. Slice tomatoes in half and also place level side down on sausage blend.

6. Add water to the skillet, cover and reduce the heat—steam for 15 mins.

7. Remove the lid and cook for another 10 minutes while sauce thickens, chopping the tomatoes with the side of your mixing spoon.

8. Boil water in a medium pot. Cook zucchini for 3-4 mins until tender. Drain pipes.

9. Serve your noodles. Garnish with chopped ramp leaves.

Nutrition: Calories: 387 Sugar: 3 g Fat: 12 g Carbohydrates: 1 g Fiber: 3 g Protein: 76 g.

15.Garlic Shrimp Zucchini Pasta.

Preparation Time: 15 minutes

Cooking time: 32 minutes

Servings: 4

Ingredients:

- 4 large zucchini (about 2 extra pounds).
- 2 tsp Salt (to salt the zucchini).
- 1/3 cup bacon oil (crispy bits make it even much better).
- 1/4 cup chopped fresh basil.
- 2 large garlic cloves, squashed.
- 1/2 cup sliced Walnuts (optional, leave out for AIP).

Directions:

1. Cut the ends off of your to fit your spiralizer.
2. Run your zucchini through your spiralizer. In a large pan, sauté your zucchini noodles with your olive oil, onion, and keep seasonings up until onion and zucchini are soft. Add your shrimp up until warmed and serve.
3. This dish features zucchini as a mock noodle, which has a sweet flavor for Italian-inspired meals.
4. Omit the walnuts to make this autoimmune recipe protocol-friendly. This recipe makes sufficient for 3-4 hearty side dish portions.

5. Alternately, you might include some barbequed steak, prawns, or chicken. Servings: 3-4.

Nutrition: Calories: 387 Sugar: 3 g Fat: 12 g Carbohydrates: 2 g Fiber: 3 g Protein: 45 g.

16. Cacio E Pepe Egg Noodles.

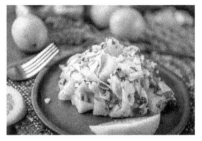

Preparation Time: 15 minutes

Cooking time: 32 minutes

Servings: 4

Ingredients:

- 4 large eggs.
- Kosher salt.
- 2 tsp. Canola oil.
- 1 tbsp. Butter.
- 1/4 c. newly grated Parmesan for serving.
- Freshly ground black pepper.

Directions:

1. Break eggs right into a tool bowl period and add salt. Blend until smooth.

2. In a nonstick skillet over medium-high heat 1 tsp oil. Add half the egg combination and twirl the frying pan to layer the bottom of the skillet with egg uniformly. Cook, continuously, until edges are formed, about 1 minute.

3. Run a spatula along edges of egg to release, then use your hands to flip the omelet gently.

4. Cook till egg is just set on the bottom, concerning 20 seconds.

5. Slide omelet onto a cutting board and also allow cool slightly for 1 min. At the same time, repeat the process with remaining oil and eggs.

6. Roll omelets up like a cigar and also cut right into 1/4- inch thick "noodles."

7. Return skillet to medium-high and melt butter. While whisking, slowly gather 1/4 cup water until incorporated. Include Parmesan and pepper, and also stir till Parmesan melts into the sauce. Include noodles and also throw to coat.

8. Season with even more pepper and also spray with more Parmesan before eating.

Nutrition: Calories: 387 Sugar: 3 g Fat: 12 g Carbohydrates: 2 g Fiber: 3 g

17.Scialatielli

Preparation Time: 15 minutes

Cooking time: 32 minutes

Servings: 4

Ingredients:

- 1 egg
- 175 g whole milk
- Basil
- 10 g, extra virgin olive oil
- 30 g grated pecorino
- 400 g durum wheat semolina

Directions:

1. Wash and dry the basil leaves and chop them finely with a knife. Pour the durum wheat in the bowl and add the beaten egg with the use of a fork.
2. Add the chopped basil, the grated pecorino and flush at room temperature after adding the milk.
3. Pour in the extra virgin olive oil and start kneading using the hand.
4. After transferring the mixture onto the pastry board, continue kneading again by hand for like 8 minutes.
5. Get homogeneous and smooth dough; leave it to rest for about 30 minutes at room temperature after wrapping it in a cling film.

6. Divide the dough into two 10s, and keep the other half, wrap it in a plastic wrap so as to prevent it from drying out because of the air. On the pastry board, work on the first part flour it with semolina using a rolling pin of about 5 mm thick.

7. After sprinkling the pastry with more semolina, drag the edges towards the center by rolling them form one side to the other till you reach the center.

8. Cut the dough into rings about 1 cm thick using a well-sharpened blade. With the help of your hands, unroll them gently. They must be like 12-15 cm long.

9. At such a point, your scialatielli are ready to be cooked in plentiful boiling and salted water for like 5 minutes.

Nutrition: Calories: 321 Sugar: 2 g Fat: 12 g Carbohydrates: 3 g Fiber: 5 g Protein: 45 g.

18. Tagliolini Fatti in Casa (Homemade Tagliolini)

Preparation time: 30 minutes

Cooking time: 5 minutes

Serves: 4

Ingredients:

- 2 medium eggs
- Semolina for pastry board
- 200 g, 00 flour

Directions:

1. Pour the flour in a bowl, add eggs and mix with a fork. Use your hands to mix until you create a homogeneous mixture.

2. Take the dough to a work surface that is lightly floured and continue working vigorously.

3. If necessary, add a little flour and work until the dough is elastic and smooth.

4. Make a ball and wrap it in a plastic wrap or put it in a food bag in a dry and cool place at room temperature for like 30 minutes.

5. When the rest time is over. Take the pasta sprinkled with little flour and divide in two parts. To avoid drying, close the film you aren't using immediately. You can pull the other using the machine or rolling pin from the lowest to the highest till you acquire a very thin sheet.

6. Put the obtained strips on a work surface, lightly floured with refilled semolina, which you can as well use to sprinkle the pasta sheets. From each sheet, make 3 rectangles and let each side dry for like 3 minutes. Without pressing, wrap the rectangles on themselves to form small rolls and use a knife to cut them into 2 mm thick strips.

7. Taking a piece of pasta, unroll the tagliolini delicately. Roll into a nest and let them dry on a clothesline or a lightly and clean floured dish towel. Continue that process till you finish all the fresh pasta.

Nutrition: Calories: 387 Sugar: 3 g Fat: 12 g Carbohydrates: 2 g Fiber: 3 g Protein: 45 g.

19. Pappardelle Fatte in Casa (Homemade Pappardelle)

Preparation time: 30 minutes

Cooking time: 10 minutes

Serves: 3

Ingredients:

- 3 eggs
- 300 g 00 flour

Directions:

1. To prepare the homemade pappardelle, put the flour in a bowl or on the work surface. Break the eggs and lightly beat them using a fork.

2. Add flour to the eggs until they have absorbed the flour and on a work surface or table, start kneading using the hand. Use the palms of your hands to work until you obtain a smooth and homogenous mixture.

3. This operation takes quite some time. To prove that all is in the right place, cut it into halves and when you see air bubbles, just know you have done a great job.

4. Make a loaf and put in closed in a plastic wrap and allow it to rest on your work surface for 15-20 minutes

5. Slightly flour the surface use a rolling pin to roll out the dough beginning from the center. Use the rolling pin to roll the dough, roll as you lightly press on the upper right and left edges. Again, roll them out and continue the same operation

until you get the thickness you desire. Allow it to dry for 10 minutes.

6. Use a little flour to sprinkle the dough and slightly fold the edges at the top and bottom, roll until it reaches at the center of the pasta circle and do it on both sides. Use a sharp knife to cut the strips 1 cm wide and unroll the strips.

7. Use the palm of your hand to roll the pappardelle a little at a time and put them on a lightly floured tray after forming a nest.

8. Cook and season them as preferred.

Nutrition: Calories: 432 Sugar: 2 g Fat: 15 g Carbohydrates: 3 g Fiber: 3 g Protein: 34 g.

20. <u>Lasagne</u>

Preparation time: 20 minutes

Cooking Time: 40 minutes

Serves: 6

Ingredients:

- 4 eggs
- 1 pinch of salt
- 400 g 00 flour

Directions::

1. Clean the work surface and make sure it is uncluttered and smooth.

2. In a classic fountain shape, pour in the flour and after you make a hole in the center, pour the shelled eggs inside and also add a pinch of salt. Use a fork to beat the eggs slowly and then move on to the more certainly and traditional method of using the fingers.

3. Incorporate the flour gradually on the edges until all ingredients are well mixed. When you get your egg pasta ball, start working on it by occasionally beating it on the lightly floured pastry board and also vigorously massaging it. This phase should last for at least 15 minutes to 1 hour. Use a damp cloth to wrap the dough and allow it to rest for 30 minutes.

4. On a floured surface, take the dough again and massage it a little more. Begin pressing it with your hands as you roll it then

to form a very thin sheet use the rolling pin, make a sheet less than a millimeter.

5. You can as well divide the dough into several portions that will be rolled out one at a given time. This will facilitate and ease this operation.

6. Depending on the size of the pan, you can now cut the pasta in rectangles of variable sizes or the shape of Lasagne. (The formats used most are 8x16 cm or 14x20)

7. You can now think about how to season the different layers after the sheet is ready.

Nutrition: Calories: 387 Sugar: 3 g Fat: 12 g Carbohydrates: 2 g Fiber: 3 g Protein: 45 g.

21.Pici Fatti a Mano (Handmade Pici)

Preparation time: 1 hour

Cooking time: 10 minutes

Serves: 4

Ingredients:

- 270 ml warm water
- 2 tbsp. olive oil
- 1 pinch of salt
- 450 g 00 flour

Directions:

1. Make the dough into a ball and put it in a plastic wrap. Let it rest for like 30 minutes after covering it with cloth. Knead it for like half a minute and take it back. On a floured surface, use a rolling pin to roll it to the thickness of 1 inch or even less. Use few oil drops to grease it and cut it into strips as large as they are high in a less or more square section.

2. Sprinkle a little wheat flour on the pastry board. Use a couple of handfuls of yellow or corn flour to prepare the tray and as you make the pici, it will help to dry them.

3. Use the fingers of your left hand to take the end of a strip and keep it raised slightly from the pastry board. Use the palm of your right hand and roll it over by rubbing and use the left hand to stretch it by pulling gently. This will enable you get a long spaghetti which you will make of fairly and uniform fine diameter.

4. When done, for it to dry, throw it on the yellow surface and move it so that it sticks. You can repeat this for all the pasta. Make sure before you throw the pici in the tray, it has been well floured to avoid them from attacking each other. After you are done making all the pici, pass them on the pastry board. This should be after removing from the tray. Spread them out and separate them from each other but always flower them well with yellow flour.

5. Allow them to dry for at least 45 minutes and a maximum of 3 hours because when fully dry, they cook well. To avoid them touching the pastry board on the same side, move them occasionally. There is no problem in case they break while you move them, just attach together the ends that have broken and continue. Do not make them very long for the first few times. Two or three palms are okay.

Nutrition: Calories: 321 Sugar: 2 g Fat: 15 g Carbohydrates: 1 g Fiber: 5 g Protein: 43 g.

22. Caprese Pasta Salad

Preparation time: 5 minutes

Cooking Time: 2 hours 30 minutes

Serving Size: 8

Ingredients:

- 1/4 cup basil (chopped)
- 2 tablespoons balsamic glaze
- 1 pound rotini (cooked)
- 1/3 cup red onion (diced)
- 1/4 cup (sun-dried) tomatoes
- 3 cups tomatoes (halved)
- 1 1/2 cups mozzarella cheese (cubed)
- Dressing
- 1 clove garlic (minced)
- salt and pepper
- 1/2 cup olive oil
- 4 tablespoons red wine vinegar

Directions::

1. In a shallow bowl, put the dressing ingredients and stir them to mix.
2. Transfer the tomatoes to the dressing mixture and wait for at least thirty minutes to marinate at ambient temperature.
3. In a medium bowl, combine the spaghetti, mozzarella, spring onion and sun-dried tomatoes.

4. Mix with the tomato/dressing combination and season with salt and pepper.

5. Before serving, put it in the fridge for at least two hours.

6. Sprinkle the balsamic glaze with the salad and sprinkle the basil on top before serving.

Nutrition: Calories 165 Fat 15, Protein 30 g, Total Carbs 5 g, Fiber 13 g

KETO CHAFFLE

23. Guacamole chaffle bites

Preparation time: 10 minutes

Cooking time: 14 minutes

Servings: 2

Ingredients:

- large turnip, cooked and mashed
- bacon slices, cooked and finely chopped
- ½ cup finely grated monterey jack cheese
- egg, beaten
- cup guacamole for topping

Directions:

1. Preheat the waffle iron.
2. Mix all the Ingredients except for the guacamole in a medium bowl.
3. Open the iron and add half of the mixture. Close and cook for 4 minutes. Open the lid, flip the chaffle and cook further until golden brown and crispy, 3 minutes.
4. Remove the chaffle onto a plate and make another in the same manner.

5. Cut each chaffle into wedges, top with the guacamole and Servings afterward.

Nutrition: Calories 311 Fats 22.52g carbs 8.29g net carbs 5.79g protein 13.62g

24. Zucchini parmesan chaffles

Preparation time: 10 minutes

Cooking time: 14 minutes

Servings: 2

Ingredients:

- cup shredded zucchini
- egg, beaten
- ½ cup finely grated parmesan cheese
- Salt and freshly ground black pepper to taste

Directions:

1. Preheat the waffle iron.
2. Put all the Ingredients in a medium bowl and mix well.
3. Open the iron and add half of the mixture. Close and cook until crispy, 7 minutes.
4. Remove the chaffle onto a plate and make another with the remaining mixture.
5. Cut each chaffle into wedges and Servings afterward.

Nutrition: Calories 138 Fats 9.07g carbs 3.81g net carbs 3.71g protein 10.02g

25. Blue cheese chaffle bites

Preparation time: 10 minutes

Cooking time: 14 minutes

Servings: 2

Ingredients:

- egg, beaten
- ½ cup finely grated parmesan cheese
- ¼ cup crumbled blue cheese
- tsp erythritol

Directions:

1. Preheat the waffle iron.
2. Mix all the Ingredients in a bowl.
3. Open the iron and add half of the mixture. Close and cook until crispy, 7 minutes.
4. Remove the chaffle onto a plate and make another with the remaining mixture.
5. Cut each chaffle into wedges and Servings afterward.

Nutrition: Calories 196 Fats 13.91g carbs 4.03g net carbs 4.03g protein 13.48g

26. Scrambled Eggs on a Spring Onion Chaffle

Servings: 4

Preparation:Time:5minutes

Cooking time 7–9 minutes

Ingredients

- Batter
- 4 eggs
- 2 cups grated mozzarella cheese
- 2 spring onions, finely chopped
- Salt and pepper to taste
- ½ teaspoon dried garlic powder
- 2 tablespoons almond flour
- 2 tablespoons coconut flour
- Other
- 2 tablespoons butter for brushing the waffle maker
- 6-8 eggs
- Salt and pepper
- teaspoon Italian spice mix
- tablespoon olive oil
- tablespoon freshly chopped parsley

Directions

1. Preheat the waffle maker.
2. Crack the eggs into a bowl and add the grated cheese.

3. Mix until just combined, then add the chopped spring onions and season with salt and pepper and dried garlic powder.

4. Stir in the almond flour and mix until everything is combined.

5. Brush the heated waffle maker with butter and add a few tablespoons of the batter.

6. Close the lid and cook for about 7–8 minutes depending on your waffle maker.

7. While the chaffles are cooking, prepare the scrambled eggs by whisking the eggs in a bowl until frothy, about 2 minutes. Season with salt and black pepper to taste and add the Italian spice mix. Whisk to blend in the spices.

8. Warm the oil in a non-stick pan over medium heat.

9. Pour the eggs in the pan and cook until eggs are set to your liking.

10. Serve each chaffle and top with some scrambled eggs. Top with freshly chopped parsley.

Nutrition (per serving) Calories 194, fat 14.7 g, carbs 5 g, sugar 0.6 g, Protein 11.1 g, sodium 191 mg

27. Ground Chicken Chaffle

Servings: 4

PreparationTime:5minutes

Cooking time 8–10 minutes

Ingredients

- Batter
- ½ pound ground chicken
- 4 eggs
- 3 tablespoons tomato sauce
- Salt and pepper to taste
- cup grated mozzarella cheese
- teaspoon dried oregano
- Other
- tablespoons butter to brush the waffle maker

Directions

1. Preheat the waffle maker.
2. Add the ground chicken, eggs and tomato sauce to a bowl and season with salt and pepper.
3. Mix everything with a fork and stir in the mozzarella cheese and dried oregano.
4. Mix again until fully combined.
5. Brush the heated waffle maker with butter and add a few tablespoons of the batter.

6. Close the lid and cook for about 8–10 minutes depending on your waffle maker.

7. Serve and enjoy.

Nutrition (per serving) Calories 246, fat 15.6 g, carbs 1.5 g, sugar 0.9 g, Protein 24.2 g, sodium 254 mg

28.   Chicken Parmesan Chaffle

Servings: 4

Preparation:Time:5minutes

Cooking time 5–7 minutes

Ingredients

- Batter
- 2 cups cooked shredded chicken breast
- 4 eggs
- 3 tablespoons tomato sauce
- ¼ cup almond flour
- Salt and pepper to taste
- ½ teaspoon dried garlic
- cup grated parmesan cheese
- teaspoon dried oregano
- tablespoons cream cheese
- cup grated mozzarella cheese
- Other
- tablespoons butter to brush the waffle maker
- ¼ cup tomato sauce

Directions

1. Preheat the waffle maker.
2. Add the chicken, eggs, almond flour, and tomato sauce to a bowl and season with salt and pepper and dried garlic.

3. Mix everything with a fork and stir in the parmesan cheese, dried oregano, and cream cheese.

4. Mix again until fully combined.

5. Brush the heated waffle maker with butter and add a few tablespoons of the grated mozzarella cheese to create the crust for the chicken parmesan chaffle.

6. Close the lid and cook for about 5–7 minutes depending on your waffle maker.

7. Repeat with the rest of the batter.

8. Serve with extra tomato sauce on top.

Nutrition (per serving) Calories 361, fat 24.3 g, carbs 5.0 g, sugar 1.8 g, Protein 32.1 g, sodium 592 mg

KETO BREAD MACHINE

29. Pumpkin Bread

Preparation Time: 50-55 minutes

Cooking Time: 0 minutes

Serving: 10 slices

Ingredients:

- 4 oz. butter
- 5 oz. erythritol
- 4 eggs
- 6 oz. pumpkin puree
- 1/3 tbsp. vanilla extract
- 12 oz. almond flour
- 4 oz. coconut flour
- 1 clove
- 1/8 tbsp. salt
- 1/8 tbsp. nutmeg
- 1/8 tbsp. ginger
- 1/3 tbsp. cinnamon
- 4 tsp. of baking powder

Directions:

1. Preheat oven to a temperature of 350 degrees Fahrenheit. Grease a nine-by-five loaf pan. Put a lining of parchment paper.

2. Take one big bowl and mix erythritol and butter until they become fluffy and light.

3. Put the eggs in it one by one. Mix well.

4. Add vanilla and pumpkin puree. Mix everything properly.

5. Take another bowl and mix coconut flour, almond flour, cinnamon, nutmeg, clove, ginger, salt, and baking powder. Break the lumps that may be there in the coconut or almond flours.

6. Then mix the dry items with the wet ones to form a batter.

7. Dispense it into the pan that you have prepared. Bake for 45 to 55 minutes.

Nutrition: Calories: 165 Carbohydrates: 5 grams Fiber: 3 grams Total fat: 14 grams Fat (saturated): 7 grams Sugar: 1 gram Protein: 5 grams

MAINS

30. Shrimp with Linguine

Preparation Time: 10 minutes

Cooking Time: 10 minutes

Servings: 4

Ingredients:

- lb Shrimp, cleaned
- lb Linguine
- tbsp Butter
- ½ cup white Wine
- ½ cup Parmesan cheese, shredded
- Garlic cloves, minced
- 1 cup Parsley, chopped
- Salt and Pepper, to taste
- ½ cup Coconut Cream, for garnish
- ½ Avocado, diced, for garnish
- tbsp fresh Dill, for garnish

Directions:

1. Melt the butter on Sauté. Stir in linguine, garlic cloves and parsley. Cook for 4 minutes until aromatic. Add shrimp and white wine; season with salt and pepper, seal the lid.

2. Select Manual and cook for 5 minutes on High pressure. When ready, quick release the pressure. Unseal and remove

the lid. Press Sauté, add the cheese and stir well until combined, for 30-40 seconds. Serve topped with the coconut cream, avocado, and dill.

Nutrition: Calories 412, Protein 48g, Net Carbs 5.6g, Fat 21g

31.Mexican Cod Fillets

Preparation Time: 10 minutes

Cooking Time: 10 minutes

Servings: 3

Ingredients:

- 3 Cod fillets
- Onion, sliced
- cups Cabbage
- Juice from 1 Lemon
- Jalapeno Pepper
- ½ tsp Oregano
- ½ tsp Cumin powder
- ½ tsp Cayenne Pepper
- tbsp Olive oil
- Salt and black Pepper to taste

Directions:

1. Heat the oil on Sauté, and add onion, cabbage, lemon juice, jalapeño pepper, cayenne pepper, cumin powder and oregano, and stir to combine. Cook for 8-10 minutes.

2. Season with salt and black pepper. Arrange the cod fillets in the sauce, using a spoon to cover each piece with some of the sauce. Seal the lid and press Manual. Cook for 5 minutes on High pressure. When ready, do a quick release and serve.

Nutrition: Calories 306, Protein 21g, Net Carbs 6.8g, Fat 19.4g

32. <u>Vegetarian Faux Stew</u>

Preparation Time: 5 minutes

Cooking Time: 25 minutes

Servings: 3

Ingredients:

- ½ cups Diced Tomatoes
- 4 cloves Garlic
- tsp Minced Ginger
- tsp Turmeric
- 1 tsp Cayenne Powder
- tsp Paprika
- Salt to taste
- 1 tsp Cumin Powder
- cups Dry Soy Curls
- 1 ½ cups Water
- tbsp Butter
- ½ cup Heavy Cream
- ¼ cup Chopped Cilantro

Directions:

1. Place the tomatoes, water, soy curls and all spices in the Instant Pot. Seal the lid, secure the pressure valve and select Manual mode on High Pressure mode for 6 minutes.

2. Once ready, do a natural pressure release for 10 minutes. Select Sauté, add the cream and butter. Stir while crushing the

tomatoes with the back of the spoon. Stir in the cilantro and serve.

Nutrition: Calories 143, Protein 4g, Net Carbs 2g, Fat 9g

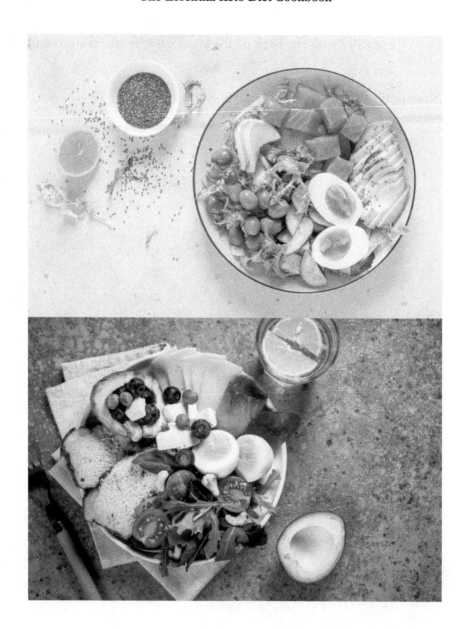

SIDES

33. Avocado and Watermelon Mix

Preparation Time: 10 minutes

Cooking Time: 0 minutes

Servings: 4

Ingredients:

- and ½ cups tomatoes, cubed
- and ½ cups watermelon, cubed
- ½ jalapeno, chopped
- A pinch of salt and black pepper
- avocado, peeled, pitted and cubed
- ½ teaspoon olive oil
- tablespoons ginger, grated
- Zest of 1 lime, grated
- teaspoons black sesame seeds
- tablespoons mint, chopped
- tablespoons lime juice

Directions:

1. In a salad bowl, combine the tomatoes with the watermelon, jalapeno, salt, pepper, avocado, oil, ginger, lime zest, black seeds, mint and lime juice, toss, divide between plates and serve as a side dish.

Nutrition: Calories: 199 Fat: 2 Fiber: 5 Carbs: 9 Protein: 5

34. <u>Celery and Chili Peppers Stir Fry</u>

Preparation Time: 10 minutes

Cooking Time: 5 minutes

Servings: 6

Ingredients:

- 2 tablespoons olive oil

- 3 chili peppers, dried and crushed

- 4 cups celery, julienned

- 2 tablespoons coconut aminos

Directions:

1. Heat up a pan with the oil at medium-high heat, add chili peppers, stir and cook them for 2 minutes.

2. Add the celery and the coconut aminos, stir, cook for 3 minutes more, divide between plates and serve as a side dish.

Nutrition: Calories: 162 Fat: 2 Fiber: 7 Carbs: 12 Protein: 7

35. Crispy Bacon and Kale

Preparation Time: 5 minutes

Cooking Time: 14 minutes

Servings: 2

Ingredients:

- ½ ounces bacon
- 4 ounces kale
- ¼ teaspoon black pepper
- Salt to taste

Directions:

1. Take a wide pot (that will be suitable for kale you'll add later), and add bacon. Cook the strips over medium heat until they become crispy. Put them aside.

2. Lower the heat, cut your kale and place it in the pot. Cook the kale on the bacon grease for 5 minutes or until it becomes wilted. Toss in some pepper and salt.

3. Slice the bacon into smaller pieces and mix it with the kale. Serve it warm!

Nutrition: Calories: 116 Total Carbs: 3,7g Fiber: 1,2g Net Carbs: 2,5g Fat: 7,7g Protein: 8,3g

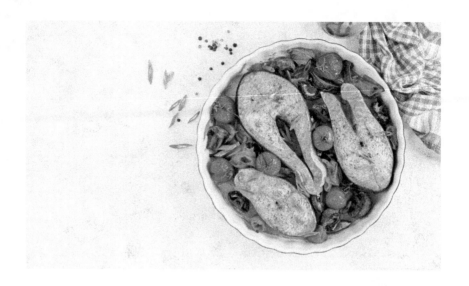

VEGETABLES

36. Sprouts and Kale Sauté

Preparation time: 5 minutes

Cooking time: 5 minutes

Servings: 2

Ingredients:

- 2 oz chopped kale
- 4 oz Brussels sprouts
- 3 tbsp chopped almonds
- tbsp white wine vinegar
- ½ tbsp avocado oil
- 1/3 tsp salt

Directions:

1. Prepare the sprout and for this, peel the leaves, starting from outside and continue peeling towards to middle until you reach the tough core.

2. Discard the core and transfer sprout leaves to a medium bowl.

3. Take a large frying pan, place it over medium heat, add oil and when hot, add sprout leaves, toss until coated with oil, and cook for 1 minute or until sauté.

4. Drizzle with vinegar, add kale, toss until mixed, and cook for 1 minute until kale leaves begin to wilt.

5. Season with salt, remove the pan from heat and garnish with almonds. Serve.

Nutrition: 210 Calories; 17.5 g Fats; 4.7 g Protein; 1.9 g Net Carb; 6 g Fiber;

37. <u>Sprouts and Bacon Plate</u>

Preparation time: 5 minutes

Cooking time: 8 minutes

Servings: 2

Ingredients:

- 4 oz Brussels sprouts
- tsp minced garlic
- slices of bacon, chopped
- tsp avocado oil
- 1/3 tsp salt
- 1/4 tsp ground black pepper

Directions:

1. Take a medium skillet pan, place it over medium heat and when hot, add bacon and cook for 3 minutes per side until crisp.
2. Add sprouts, add oil, toss until mixed and cook for 10 minutes until thoroughly cooked.
3. Stir in garlic, season with salt and black pepper and continue cooking for 1 minute.
4. Serve.

Nutrition: 145 Calories; 11.2 g Fats; 5.4 g Protein; 3.2 g Net Carb; 2.2 g Fiber;

38.   <u>Salad in Jar</u>

Preparation time: 5 minutes

Cooking time: 0 minutes

Servings: 2

Ingredients:

- 2 oz chopped kale
- scallion, chopped
- avocado, pitted, chopped
- Roma tomato, chopped
- 4 slices of beef roast, diced
- ½ cup mayonnaise

Directions:

1. Take two mason jars, place kale evenly at the bottom and then top with kale, scallion, avocado, and tomato.
2. Top with beef and serve each jar with ¼ cup mayonnaise.

Nutrition: 438 Calories; 38 g Fats; 13.5 g Protein; 5.5 g Net Carb; 8.5 g Fiber;

39.   Cauliflower Cups

Preparation Time: 5 minutes

Cooking Time: 30 minutes

Servings: 6

Ingredients:

- ½ cups cauliflower rice
- ¼ cup diced onion
- ½ cup shredded pepper jack cheese
- ½ tsp dried oregano
- ½ tsp dried basil
- ½ tsp salt
- large egg, lightly beaten

Directions:

1. Preheat the oven to 350F.
2. Put and mix all ingredients in a bowl
3. Scoop mixture into the wells of a mini muffin tin and pack lightly.
4. Bake for 30 minutes.
5. Cool and serve.

Nutrition: Calories 60 Fat 3.9g Carbs 1.8g Protein 4.3g

SOUPS AND STEWS

40. Broccoli Cheddar Soup

Preparation Time: 5 minutes

Cooking Time: 35 minutes

Servings: 6

Ingredients:

- ⅓ cup olive oil
- large yellow onion, chopped
- garlic cloves, minced
- ⅓ cup all-purpose flour
- cups Classic Vegetable Broth
- cups whole milk
- Salt
- Black pepper
- teaspoon mustard powder
- ⅛ teaspoon allspice
- ⅛ teaspoon nutmeg
- cups finely chopped broccoli florets
- large carrots, peeled and grated
- cups shredded sharp cheddar cheese

Directions:

1. Heat the olive oil in a large stockpot or Dutch oven over medium heat. Add the onion and cook until translucent, about 2 minutes. Add the garlic and cook 1 minute more. Whisk in the flour and create a simple roux. Allow to cook until golden brown, 2 to 3 minutes.

2. Reduce the heat to medium-low and add the broth and milk, whisking to dissolve the roux into the liquid. Season with salt and pepper, then add the mustard powder, allspice, and nutmeg.

3. Add the broccoli and carrots and gently simmer for 15 to 20 minutes, until the broccoli is tender. Add the cheese, reserving a small amount for topping. Transfer to serving bowls, garnish with the reserved cheese, and serve immediately.

Nutrition: Calories: 390 Fat: 27g Protein: 13g Cholesterol: 50mg Sodium: 400mg Carbohydrates: 20g Fiber: 3g

41. Maltese Fish Soup

Preparation Time: 10 minutes

Cooking Time: 10 minutes

Servings: 4

Ingredients:

- whole small fish, cleaned and sliced into 4 pieces
- 8 cups water
- tbsp. olive oil
- 6 tomatoes, sliced
- lemons (one for juice, one for garnish)
- onion, chopped
- garlic cloves, chopped
- bay leaf
- 1 tbsp. fresh mint, chopped
- ¼ cup fresh parsley, chopped
- Salt and pepper to taste

Directions:

1. Add the olive oil to the instant pot bowl and sauté the onions and garlic for 3 minutes.
2. Add in the fish, tomatoes, mint, bay leaf, and water.
3. Secure the lid, seal the vent, and cook on "HIGH" pressure for 7 minutes.

4. Do a quick release and remove the fish and the bay leaf from the pot. Once it has cooled, remove the head, skin, tail, and bones.

5. Return the fish to the pot. Stir.

6. Season with salt and pepper, and squeeze 1 lemon on top.

7. Serve hot and garnish with parsley and lemon wedges.

Nutrition: Calories: 226 Kcal Fat: 12 g Proteins: 40 g Net carbs: 9 g

DRESSING AND SAUCES

42. Marinara Sauce

Preparation Time: 10 minutes

Cooking Time: 5 minutes

Servings: 12

Ingredients:

- 2 tablespoons olive oil
- garlic clove
- teaspoons onion flakes
- teaspoons fresh thyme, finely chopped
- 2 teaspoons fresh oregano, finely chopped
- 24 ounces tomato puree
- tablespoon balsamic vinegar
- teaspoons Erythritol
- Salt and ground black pepper, as required
- tablespoons fresh parsley, finely chopped

Directions:

1. Warm the oil in a medium pan at medium-low heat and sauté the garlic, onion flakes, thyme, and oregano for about 3 minutes.

2. Stir in the tomato puree, vinegar, Erythritol, salt, and black pepper and bring to a gentle simmer.

3. Remove the pan of sauce from heat and stir in the parsley.

4. Place at room temperature to cool completely before serving.

5. You can preserve this sauce in the refrigerator by placing it into an airtight container.

Nutrition: Calories: 36 Net Carbs: 3.6g Carbohydrate: 4.7g Fiber: 1.1g Protein: 0.9g Fat: 2g Sugar: 2.3g Sodium: 168mg

43. Spinach Sauce with Milk

Preparation Time: 20 minutes

Cooking Time: 5 minutes

Servings: 4

Ingredients:

- 4 cups spinach, chopped
- 2 tbsp. almond flour
- ½ tsp agar powder
- small onion, finely chopped
- garlic cloves, crushed
- ½ cup whole milk
- ¼ cup sour cream
- Spices:
- ½ tsp white pepper
- ½ tsp sea salt

Directions:

1. Rinse well the spinach on the cold running water and drain in a large colander. Put in the pot and add butter. Press the "Saute" button then stir. Cook until spinach has wilted.

2. Put onions and garlic. Dust with salt and pepper and cook for 2 minutes, stirring constantly.

3. Finally, pour in the milk and add sour cream, almond flour, and agar powder. Stir well and bring it to a boil. Cook for 2 minutes, stirring constantly.

Nutrition: Calories 123 Total Fats: 7.8g Net Carbs: 7.3g Protein: 5.3g Fiber: 1.6g

44. Sour Garlic Sauce

Preparation Time: 10 minutes

Cooking Time: 5 minutes

Servings: 4

Ingredients:

- 3 garlic cloves, crushed
- ½ cup of milk
- tbsp. almond flour
- tbsp. butter
- tsp apple cider vinegar
- Spices:
- ¼ tsp dried thyme
- ¼ tsp garlic powder

Directions:

1. Grease the inner pot with butter and press the "Saute" button. Heat up and add garlic. Sprinkle with thyme and garlic powder.

2. Cook for at least 1 minute and then add milk. Drizzle with apple cider vinegar and bring it to a boil.

3. Press the "Cancel" button and remove it from the pot. Serve with meat.

Nutrition: Calories 121 Total Fats: 9.3g Net Carbs: 5.6g Protein: 4g Fiber: 0.4g

DESSERT

45. <u>Sugar-Free Lemon Bars</u>

Preparation Time: 15 minutes

Cooking Time: 45 minutes

Servings: 8

Ingredients:

- ½ cup butter, melted
- 1¾ cup almond flour, divided
- cup powdered erythritol, divided
- medium-size lemons
- large eggs

Directions:

1. Prepare the parchment paper and baking tray. Combine butter, 1 cup of almond flour, ¼ cup of erythritol, and salt. Stir well. Place the mix on the baking sheet, press a little and put it into the oven (preheated to 350°F). Cook for about 20 minutes. Then set aside to let it cool.

2. Zest 1 lemon and juice all of the lemons in a bowl. Add the eggs, ¾ cup of erythritol, ¾ cup of almond flour, and salt. Stir together to create the filling. Pour it on top of the cake and

cook for 25 minutes. Cut into small pieces and serve with lemon slices.

Nutrition: Carbohydrates – 4 g Fat – 26 g Protein – 8 g Calories – 272

46.   <u>Creamy Hot Chocolate</u>

Preparation Time: 5 minutes

Cooking Time: 5 minutes

Servings: 4

Ingredients:

- 6 oz. dark chocolate, chopped
- ½ cup unsweetened almond milk
- ½ cup heavy cream
- Tbsp. Erythritol
- ½ tsp vanilla extract

Directions:

1. Combine the almond milk, erythritol, and cream in a small saucepan. Heat it (choose medium heat and cook for 1-2 minutes).

2. Add vanilla extract and chocolate. Stir continuously until the chocolate melts.

3. Pour into cups and serve.

Nutrition: Carbohydrates – 4 g Fat – 18 g Protein – 2 g Calories – 193

47. <u>Delicious Coffee Ice Cream</u>

Preparation Time: 10 minutes

Cooking Time: 5 minutes

Servings: 1

Ingredients:

- 6 ounces coconut cream, frozen into ice cubes
- ripe avocado, diced and frozen
- ½ cup coffee expresso
- Tbsp. sweetener
- tsp vanilla extract
- Tbsp. water
- Coffee beans

Directions:

1. Take out the frozen coconut cubes and avocado from the fridge. Slightly melt them for 5-10 minutes.

2. Add the sweetener, coffee expresso, and vanilla extract to the coconut-avocado mix and whisk with an immersion blender until it becomes creamy (for about 1 minute). Pour in the water and blend for 30 seconds.

3. Top with coffee beans and enjoy!

Nutrition: Carbohydrates – 20.5 g Fat – 61 g Protein – 6.3 g Calories – 596

48. Fatty Bombs with Cinnamon and Cardamom

Preparation Time: 10 minutes

Cooking Time: 35 minutes

Servings: 10

Ingredients:

- ½ cup unsweetened coconut, shredded
- 3 oz unsalted butter
- ¼ tsp ground green cinnamon
- ¼ ground cardamom
- ½ tsp vanilla extract

Directions:

1. Roast the unsweetened coconut (choose medium-high heat) until it begins to turn lightly brown.
2. Combine the room-temperature butter, half of the shredded coconut, cinnamon, cardamom, and vanilla extract in a separate dish. Cool the mix in the fridge for about 5-10 minutes.
3. Form small balls and cover them with the remaining shredded coconut.
4. Cool the balls in the fridge for about 10-15 minutes.

Nutrition: Carbohydrates – 0.4 g Fat – 10 g Protein – 0.4 g Calories – 90

49.   <u>Easy Peanut Butter Cups</u>

Preparation Time: 10 minutes

Cooking Time: 1 hour 35 minutes

Servings: 12 servings

Ingredients:

- 1/2 cup peanut butter
- 1/4 cup butter
- 3 oz. cacao butter, chopped
- 1/3 cup powdered swerve sweetener
- 1/2 tsp vanilla extract
- 4 oz. sugar free dark chocolate

Direction:

1. Line a muffin tin with parchment paper or cupcake liners.
2. Using low heat, melt the peanut butter, butter, and cacao butter in a saucepan. Stir them until completely combined.
3. Add the vanilla and sweetener until there are no more lumps.
4. Carefully place the mixture in the muffin cups.
5. Refrigerate it until firm
6. Put chocolate in a bowl and set the bowl in boiling water. This is done to avoid direct contact with the heat. Stir the chocolate until completely melted.

7. Take the muffin out of the fridge and drizzle in the chocolate on top. Put it back again in the fridge to firm it up. This should take 15 minutes to finish.

8. Store and serve when needed.

Nutrition: Calories: 200kFat: 19gCarbohydrates: 6gProtein: 2.9gFiber: 3.6g

50.   <u>Raspberry Mousse</u>

Preparation Time: 10 minutes

Cooking Time: 4 hours

Servings: 8

Ingredients:

- 3 oz. fresh raspberry
- 2 cups heavy whipping cream
- 2 oz. pecans, chopped
- ¼ tsp vanilla extract
- ½ lemon, the zest

Directions:

1. Pour the whipping cream into the dish and blend until it becomes soft.
2. Put the lemon zest and vanilla into the dish and mix thoroughly.
3. Put the raspberries and nuts into the cream mix and stir well.
4. Cover the dish with plastic wrap and put it in the fridge for 3 hours.
5. Top with raspberries and serve.

Nutrition: Carbohydrates – 3 g Fat – 26 g Protein – 2 g Calories – 255

CONCLUSION

K eto can be a great option for people looking to shed extra weight that is stored in their bodies as fat. Ketosis is the process of the body using fats instead of glucose for energy. The liver can take fats and break them down into ketones, which can be used by both the body and the brain as a fuel source. To get the body away from using sugars, however, a person has to severely limit the amount and type of carbs they consume so the body can burn through its glucose stores and start working on the fat stores. This is why it can be so important to stay diligent on the diet once started; otherwise, a person might not see their desired results.

For people who are ready to dedicate themselves 100% to the keto diet, there are various forms of it that can match any person's lifestyle and goals. The standard keto option is best for people trying the diet for the first time because it can be the quickest way to get into ketosis and reap the immediate benefits. There are also cyclical and targeted keto for people who might not be willing to follow the strict diet every day. These options give people an opportunity to consume carbs on certain days based on their own personal plans.

There are many benefits to starting the keto diet beyond just losing weight. Keto can also help people improve their heart health by reducing bad fats and forcing the body to work through fats it has stored, possibly in dangerous places like arteries. It can also help people with certain types of epilepsy reduce seizures by switching the brain onto ketone power. Keto can also help women with PCOS regain their health by promoting weight loss and helping to balance their hormones, which can be a cause of the condition. It can even help clear up acne in some people by reducing blood sugar, which can improve skin conditions.

It is not difficult to switch to and stick to a Keto diet. What is actually difficult is adhering to strict rules and guidelines. As long as you maintain the Fats : Protein : Carbs ratio, you'll lose weight fast. It's a no-brainer. And quite unbecoming that many have deviated from this core principle of the Keto diet. The simple formula is to increase the fat and protein content in your meals and snacks while reducing your carb intake. You must restrict your carb intake to reach and remain in Ketosis. Different people achieve Ketosis with varying amounts of carb intake. Generally, it is easy to reach and stay in Ketosis when you decrease your carb intake to not more than 20grams.

Keeping keto long term can seem difficult for beginners who are just getting used to the mechanics of the diet, but it is not so difficult once they are acclimated to the keto lifestyle. Planning out meals and snacks can help people keep up keto longer because it takes some of the work and thinking out of dieting. A person can simply grab what they need and go. And if the standard keto doesn't work for someone long term, they can refer to the other keto styles to find one that will work for them beyond the initial diet.

CPSIA information can be obtained
at www.ICGtesting.com
Printed in the USA
BVHW040735100321
602119BV00006BA/1271